Nutraceuticals in Human Health

About the series 'Books for the Concerned Citizen'

Leveraging the diverse expertise of its members in the subject domains and in publishing, the TERI Alumni Association is publishing a series of books on topics related to energy, resources, and the environment. The idea is to share information and, even more important, critical insights and understanding, with citizens who are keen to know more about some of the critical issues facing society and the world today but are lost in the deluge of information.

Our target audience is educated adults who are concerned about topical issues but lack the understanding to make sense of what they read or watch in the mass media—the series aims to equip them with conceptual tools and essential information not only to enrich their understanding but also to encourage them to act and thereby, albeit indirectly, further the UN Sustainable Development Goals.

The topics to be covered in the series and their respective subject-matter-specialist authors are listed below.

- **Rooftop solar***: Suneel Deambi and Shirish Garud
- **Coal***: Rakesh Kacker
- **Sustainable buildings***: Mili Majumdar and Minni Sastry
- **Nutraceuticals**: Mayurika Goel
- **Electricity**: Sanjeev S Ahluwalia
- **Public transport**: Shri Prakash and Sharif Qamar
- **Energy efficiency**: Ajay Mathur and Leher Thadani
- **Climate change**: Manish Shrivastava

   *already published and available for purchase

The publication of this series is financially supported by the Shakti Sustainable Energy Foundation. All books, being printed and marketed by TERI, will be published latest October 2022.

Nutraceuticals in Human Health

Mayurika Goel

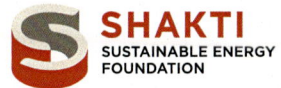 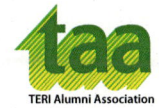

© TERI Alumni Association 2022

ISBN: 978-93-94657-05-2

Suggested citation
Goel M. 2022. *Nutraceuticals in Human Health.*
New Delhi: TERI Alumni Association. 42 pp.

TERI Alumni Association
Administrative Wing, TERI
Darbari Seth Block (ground floor)
Habitat Place
Lodhi Road
New Delhi – 110 003

Price Rs 299/-. For sales queries, please contact us at
    Nand K Yadav, Assistant Manager - Sales
    The Energy and Resources Institute (TERI Press)
    Darbari Seth Block, Habitat Place
    Lodhi Road, New Delhi – 110 003

    +91 97 173 56537 or +91 (0) 11 7110 2100 or 2468 2100
    nandkumar.yadav@teri.res.in or teripress@teri.res.in
    Fax +91 2468 2144 or 2468 2145

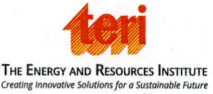

For more information, contact
Mayurika Goel (mayurikagoel@gmail.com)

CONTENTS

Foreword	vii
Preface	ix
Food is medicine: introducing nutraceuticals	1
Function of food nutrients: the balanced diet	2
Indian diet and changes in lifestyle	3
Various definitions of nutraceuticals	6
Nutraceuticals: an umbrella term	9
Some terms under the Food Safety and Standards Act	14
Sources of nutraceuticals	17
What is in our food supplements	19
Consumer awareness and regulation	18
Labelling categories and claims	18
How to read a label	22
Regulations and false claims	23
Marketing gimmicks versus realities	24
Pharmaceuticals versus nutraceuticals	25
Current market space for nutraceuticals	26
Global trends in a nutshell	27
Indian scenario	28
Major growth drivers of nutraceuticals market	31
Restorative concluding remarks	34
Consuming nutraceuticals: frequently asked questions	35
Honest Abe's valuable advice	38
Challenges for nutraceuticals	39
Final remarks: individual-centric approach to nutraceuticals	40
Bibliography	41
Some useful websites	42

FOREWORD

Health and dietary supplements, nutraceuticals, functional foods, probiotics, etc. are terms that can be quite confusing to a layperson. In addition, the terms traditional foods, functional foods, and nutraceuticals are often used interchangeably, and there is scope for miscommunication if the underlying differences among all food categories are not properly understood. I was introduced to these terms first during my stint as Director, MOFPI (Ministry of Food Processing Industries) and then as Director (Codex) in the FSSAI (Food Safety and Standards Authority of India), in which I was closely associated with the work of the Scientific Panel on Functional Foods, Nutraceuticals, Dietetic Products and other Similar Products. The standards authority also brought out the first regulations on the subject in 2016. I came to know that our good old curd or yogurt is not only a functional food but also falls in the category of probiotics! I also learnt that *chyavanprash,* which has been used for ages in India, is another example of functional foods.

The demand for nutritious diets was a major factor driving the growth of the global nutraceutical market. However, in the wake of the COVID-19 pandemic, consumers began focusing on preventive measures and overall well-being, and the demand for these products saw a further uptick. At the same time, a fine line separates nutraceuticals, health supplements, etc. from drugs, and consumers need to be aware of the distinction. Against this background, it is most opportune that this book is being brought out. It will demystify these terms and also give consumers some guidance on what to look for in reading the labels, when they buy these products. Reading product labels while buying these products is very important, because these labels are like windows: they let us peek and see what lies inside.

The author of the book, Dr Mayurika Goel, has an excellent scientific grounding as an accomplished scientist working in this area. She brings the rigour of scientific writing in an easy-to-understand manner for the common consumer intending to buy these products.

I have been following the developments in this field, and this book has renewed my interest in the subject. The global regulatory guidelines aim at regulating various aspects of the nutraceutical and dietary supplements market, focusing on their manufacture, testing, registration, labelling, and sale and to ensure safety and quality of the product. This book in a greatly simplified manner touches upon some of these facets from Indian regulatory perspective.

I am sure the concerned citizens of the country will find the book useful and it will help them in making informed decisions while buying nutraceuticals and related products. I wish the book and its author success.

June 2022

Dr Vinod Kotwal
Former Director, MoFPI and FSSAI

PREFACE

I take this opportunity to express my sincere gratitude and indebtedness to Dr Vibha Dhawan, Director General, TERI, for providing me the opportunity of being part of the 'Concerned Citizen' series of books and for introducing me to the team that managed the series. Her constant support and encouragement were invaluable throughout the journey of writing this book.

I owe a big thanks to the coordinator of the series and the president of TAA, Mr Rakesh Kacker, for being a constant source of motivation and push to write the book on time. He advised on all the aspects of the book, starting from writing the first chapter to getting it in the shape of a published book, and he was always available to help even with any minor problem related to the book. He also introduced me to Dr Vinod Kotwal, former director of FSSAI and MOFPI, who not only contributed the foreword to this book but also guided me whenever I needed her guidance and gave me the benefit of her vast and deep knowledge of the subject. I would like to express my admiration for the insightful discussions we had and the efforts she has put in to make this a better book. Many thanks are also due to Ms Mehak Kaur, my student from the TERI School of Advanced Studies, who gave me a lot of material and some very creative suggestions for improving the overall presentation of the book, and to my friend Dr Soma Patnaik, Scientist, THSTI, the Translational Health Science and Technology Institute, for lending a helping hand during the initial phase of writing and always inspiring me with her words of encouragement.

I must acknowledge the constructive suggestions and careful editing suggested by TAA members, Mr Yateendra Joshi and Mr P K Jayanthan for making the read interesting and presentable. I am also thankful to my colleagues Ms Anupama Jauhary, Mr Rajiv Sharma, and Mr Vijay Nipane of TERI Press for providing all the help to prepare the infographics and for seeing the book through the press.

Finally, I wish to express my gratitude to my father, Mr K C Goel, for encouraging me to push boundaries and teaching me that there are no shortcuts in life except hard work. Words could never do justice in expressing special thanks to my husband, Mr Vikas Bansal, for providing me constant support and keeping my spirits high throughout the journey.

The food industry has gone through major breakthroughs in recent years. These changes are in response to consumer demand for food products balanced in calories and made with nutritional ingredients and natural additives. Today, given the change in dietary habits, increased awareness on account of a rapidly growing middle class, and consumer preferences for healthy choices especially after the covid-19 pandemic, food alone is unable to meet the nutritional needs of the human body fully. The nutraceutical industry, which is an integral part of preventive health care, is undergoing a transformation in India. India's traditional herbs and preparations have withstood the test of time and Indian food and its ingredients are competitive in the global arena of preventive health care. The regulatory framework in the sector has also evolved, encompassing, among others, such areas as research, production, processing, labelling, and packaging. In these times, when awareness of food on the table is all the more important, this book on different aspects of nutraceuticals is expected to help the general reader to understand them better.

Food is medicine: introducing nutraceuticals

Let food be thy medicine, and medicine be thy food.

Hippocrates

The world's wisdom on health is captured by the above prophetic statement from the father of Western medicine, Hippocrates. This statement on food reflects the critical importance of appropriate food for health and its therapeutic benefits. Food is fundamental to our existence. Through the centuries, we have acquired a wealth of information about the use of food to ensure the growth of children and the young, to maintain good health all through our life, to meet the special needs of pregnancy and lactation, and to recover from illness. A large part of our food heritage is scientifically beneficial and needs to be retained; however, some aspects may need to be modified in view of the changes in our lifestyle.

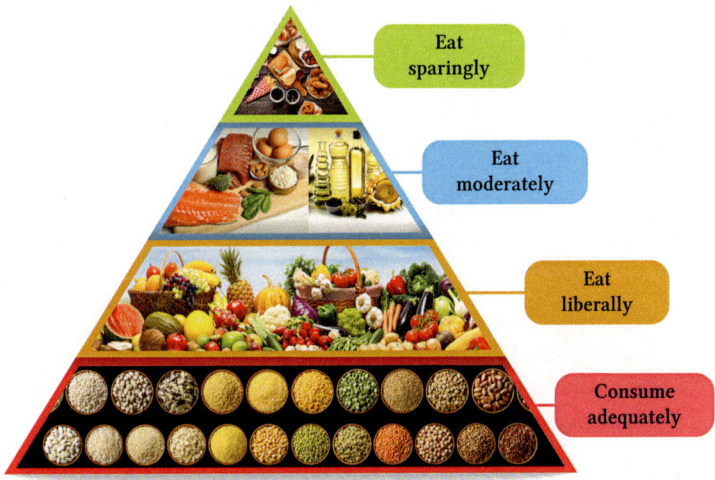

Figure 1 **Food pyramid to understand how to make a meal plan. Modified from website** (https://www.nin.res.in/downloads/DietaryGuidelines for NINwebsite.pdf)

Function of food nutrients: the balanced diet

Food provides nutrients and thus forms the basis of nutrition. Nutrients are the components of food that are required by the body in adequate amounts in order to grow, reproduce, and lead a normal, healthy life. Each nutrient has its own function, but the various nutrients must act in unison for effective action. The term usually used for these combined nutrients is 'balanced diet'. A balanced diet is that which contains a variety of foods in such quantities and proportions that the body's need for all nutrients is adequately met for maintaining health, vitality, and general well-being and also makes a small provision for extra nutrients to withstand short durations during which food may be either unavailable or in short supply (Figure 1). Unbalanced diet, on the other hand, does not have enough quantities or the correct ratio of all the nutrients required by an individual—the main difference between the two, a balanced diet and an unbalanced diet, being in the composition of nutrients each supplies. Enter nutrition, the science of food and its relationship to health. Nutrition gives us approximate but useful information on what to eat, how much to eat, and what can happen if we eat too much or too little of any particular food. The main components of a balanced diet are summarized in Table 1 and Figure 2.

According to the World Health Organization, a healthy diet for adults consists of the following components.

- Fruits, vegetables, legumes (e.g., lentils, beans), nuts and whole grains (e.g., unprocessed maize, millet, oats, wheat, brown rice).
- At least 400 grams (5 portions) of fruits and vegetables a day. Potatoes, sweet potatoes, cassava and other starchy roots are not classified as fruits or vegetables.
- Unsaturated fats (e.g., found in fish, avocado, nuts, sunflower, canola and olive oils) are preferable to saturated fats (e.g., found in fatty meat, butter, palm and coconut oil, cream, cheese, ghee and lard). Industrial trans fats (found in processed food, fast food,

snack food, fried food, frozen pizza, pies, cookies, margarines and spreads) are not part of a healthy diet.
o Less than 5 grams of iodized salt (equivalent to approximately 1 teaspoon) per day.

Table 1 Main components of a balanced diet

Component	Major function	Found in
Carbohydrates	Energy, growth, sustenance	Rice, wheat, and other grains, sweet potato, potato, corn, fresh fruits, jaggery, honey, dates, jam
Fats	Energy storage	Mustard, olive, almond, coconut, and sunflower oil, nuts, butter, fish, full-cream milk
Proteins	Building blocks: growth and repair	Lentils, nuts, soyabean, chicken, fish, milk and other dairy products
Minerals	Structural parts of bones, tissues, organs; regulation of processes	Green leafy vegetables, fruits, dried or sweet pickled fruits, berries, nuts, fish, tomato, beans, sprouts, milk, etc.
Vitamins	Vital processes	Citrus fruits, orange and dark green vegetables, amla, apple, meat, fish, eggs, poultry, soyabean
Water	Maintenance of body temperature	Cucumber, watermelon, tomatoes, lettuce, peaches, apples

Indian diet and changes in lifestyle

India's economy is driven by agriculture, which is the key sector for generating employment opportunities for the vast majority of the country's population, about 70% of which depends on agriculture for livelihood. Food habits of most Indians were based on carbohydrates to provide energy. However, our lifestyle has changed drastically over the last few decades as people began moving to cities for employment opportunities. With increase in computerization, the jobs available to the educated demand little manual labour—the only time the white-collar workers are physically active is either when they are forced to or when they decide to incorporate physical exercise into their daily routine voluntarily. With the massive increase in population that India witnessed towards the later years of the 20th century, the competition for employment increased markedly in the first decades of the 21st century, resulting in greater stress among the working class and students. Today, we experience many new ailments that have spawned by drastic changes in our way of life and by increased stress. A majority of these ailments are the 'gifts' of increasing computerization and industrialization involving a desk job work culture or the 9-to-5 routine that has people glued to their computers for more than 8 hours and at least 5 days a week. This change in lifestyle has led to a rapid increase in diabetes, hypertension, high cholesterol, and heart diseases, the polycystic ovary syndrome or polycystic ovary disease, obesity, and many more. But how did this actually happen?

> Box **1** Glossary
> **Food** is that which nourishes the body.
>
> **Nutrition** is the food at work inside the body.
>
> **Health** refers to the condition of the body.
>
> **Good** health implies freedom from diseases along with the physical, mental and emotional fitness.

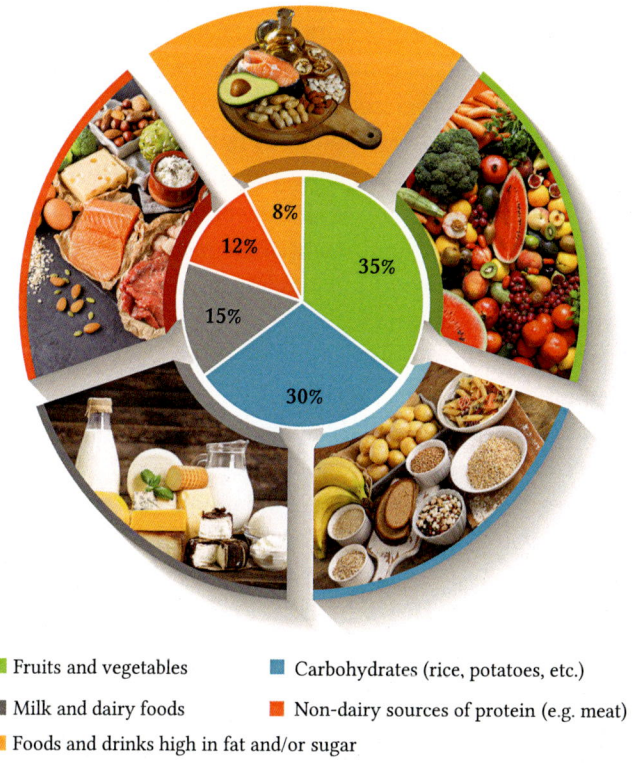

- Fruits and vegetables
- Carbohydrates (rice, potatoes, etc.)
- Milk and dairy foods
- Non-dairy sources of protein (e.g. meat)
- Foods and drinks high in fat and/or sugar

Figure **2** A balanced diet

    The fast-paced life in cities and the continued mental stress imposed by such a life led people to switch to ready-to-cook or ready-to-eat foods from the conventional diet, which used to supply all required nutrients. It is now increasingly difficult to have a balanced diet, which comprises vegetables, whole grains, milk, protein-rich pulses or meat on a daily basis to fulfil the basic dietary requirements with the recommended nutrient intake. The hustle culture does not allow us to spend time to ensure our health and well-being. Home-cooked food has now been replaced with ready-to-eat or fast foods such as noodles, pizzas, and burgers often accompanied by soft drinks. This combination, referred to as

HFSS (high in fat, sugar and salt), and the highly processed foods, have smaller amounts of proteins, dietary fibre, macronutrients, micronutrients, and other minerals and are loaded with free sugars, saturated fatty acids, and trans fatty acids. Some of these foods also contain artificial colours and additives, which might be harmful to people and to the environment. The more frequently seen deficiencies are of such essential vitamins as folic acid or riboflavin; minerals such as calcium, magnesium, iron, and zinc; and essential amino acids. Current statistics by the National Nutrition Monitoring Bureau in its reports on urban and rural populations show that the proportion of people who consume less nutritious food is far greater than what we imagine it to be. The question therefore is this: How can we be sure that we are taking the required amount of nutrients? And if not, what are the options to cover the gap?

Various definitions of nutraceuticals

Nutraceuticals is the buzz word these days, especially after the COVID-19 outbreak during which we really started to take our body and its needs seriously. *Nutraceutical* is a combination of *nutritional* and *pharmaceutical*. The concept of nutraceuticals is not entirely new, although it has evolved considerably over the years. In the early 1900s, food manufacturers in the United States began adding iodine to salt in an effort to prevent goitre, representing one of the first attempts at creating a functional component through fortification. According to the FDA (U S Food and Drug Administration), a nutraceutical is any substance that is a food or part of a food that has medicinal or health benefits. Nutraceuticals may help prevent or treat diseases. These products can be single nutrients such as vitamin C or they can be dietary supplements such as a combination of multiple vitamins and minerals. A nutraceutical can also be a genetically engineered designer food. Today researchers have identified hundreds of compounds with functional qualities and continue to make new discoveries related to the complex benefits of phytochemicals (non-nutritive plant chemicals that have protective or disease-preventive properties) in foods. Nutraceuticals can also be added to processed foods such as cereals fortified with iron. Even sports drinks with electrolytes are claimed to contain nutraceuticals. Nutraceuticals have begun to attract many consumers who are increasingly concerned about wellness, the cost of health care, and strict food laws affecting labels on food packages and product claims. Also, consumer interest in the relationship between diet and health has increased the demand for information on nutraceuticals.

> Box 2 Nutraceuticals defined
> **Food or part of food** that provides medical or health benefits, including the prevention and/or treatment of a disease
> **A diet supplement** that delivers a concentrated form of a biologically active component of food in a non-food matrix to enhance health
> **Any substance** that is a food or a part of a food and is able to induce medical and health benefits, including the prevention and treatment of disease
> **A foodstuff** (as a fortified food or dietary supplement) that provides health benefits in addition to its basic nutritional value
> Nutritional products that provide health and medical benefits, including the prevention and treatment of disease

Box 3 Food Safety and Standards Authority of India on nutraceuticals

The sets globally benchmarked standards for food and encourages the food industry to adapt good manufacturing practices. Here is an excerpt from Section 22 (1) of the Indian Food Safety and Standards Act, 2006.

(1) "foods for special dietary uses or functional foods or nutraceuticals or health supplements" means:

    (a) foods which are specially processed or formulated to satisfy particular dietary requirements which exist because of a particular physical or physiological condition or specific diseases and disorders and which are presented as such, wherein the composition of these foodstuffs must differ significantly from the composition of ordinary foods of comparable nature, if such ordinary foods exist, and may contain one or more of the following ingredients, namely: -

        (i) plants or botanicals or their parts in the form of powder, concentrate or extract in water, ethyl alcohol or hydro alcoholic extract, single or in combination;

        (ii) minerals or vitamins or proteins or metals or their compounds or amino acids (in amounts not exceeding the Recommended Daily Allowance for Indians) or enzymes (within permissible limits);

        (iii) substances from animal origin;

        (iv) a dietary substance for use by human beings to supplement the diet by increasing the total dietary intake

    (b)

        (i) a product that is labelled as a "Food for special dietary uses or functional foods or nutraceuticals or health supplements or similar such foods" which is not represented for use as a conventional food and whereby such products may be formulated in the form of powders, granules, tablets, capsules, liquids, jelly and other dosage forms but not parenteral, and are meant for oral administration;

(ii) such product does not include a drug as defined in clause (b) and ayurvedic, sidha and unani drugs as defined in clauses (a) and (h) of section 3 of the Drugs and Cosmetics Act, 1940 (23 of 1940) and rules made there under;

(iii) does not claim to cure or mitigate any specific disease, disorder or condition (except for certain health benefit or such promotion claims) as may be permitted by the regulations made under this Act;

(iv) does not include a narcotic drug or a psychotropic substance as defined in the Schedule of the Narcotic Drugs and Psychotropic Substances Act, 1985 (61 of 1985) and rules made there under and substances listed in Schedules E and E(1) of the Drugs and Cosmetics Rules, 1945.

Nutraceuticals: an umbrella term

To keep the body in good health is a duty . . . otherwise we shall not be able to keep our mind strong and clear.

Buddha

Just as food comes in all shapes and sizes with endless flavours and varieties, nutraceuticals also have quite a number of names and types under them, and clear-cut demarcations are yet to be identified in classifying them. The term 'nutraceutical' in itself is an umbrella term covering the entire range between 'conventional foods' and 'pharmacologically defined drugs' (Figure 3). Nutraceuticals are taken from natural sources and then go through various levels of processing before they reach our table. It would be best to understand nutraceuticals on the basis of what they are made of, why they are needed, when they are to be taken.

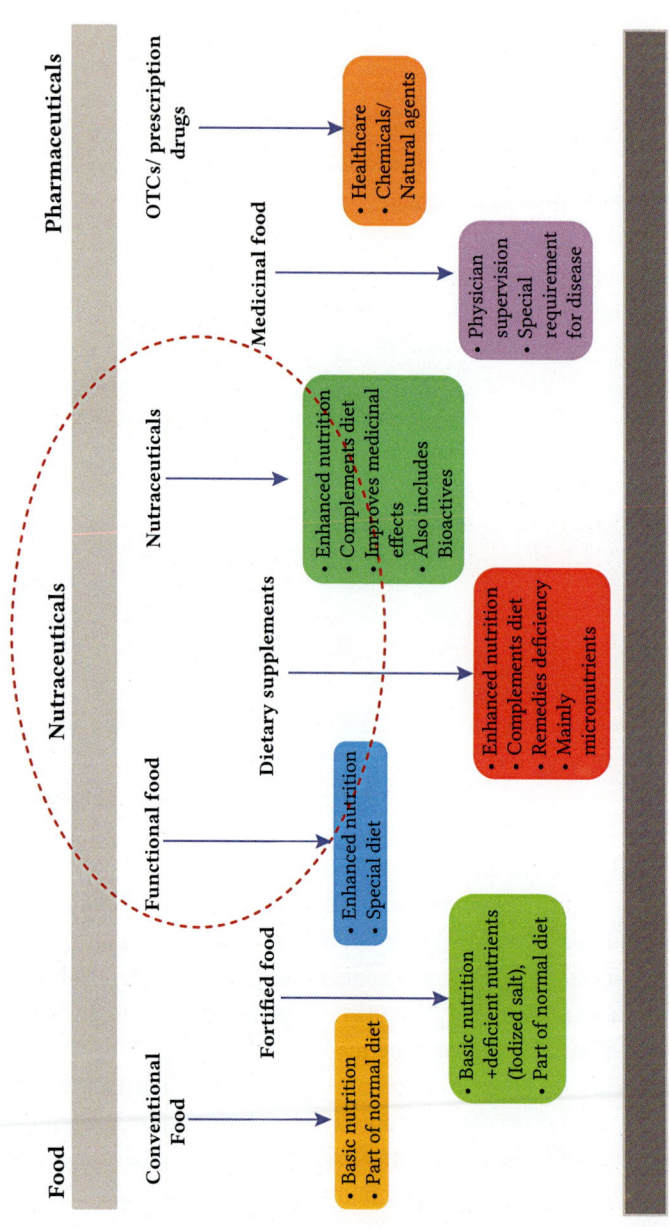

Figure 3 The umbrella term 'nutraceuticals'

Conventional food is the staple food (such as rice, wheat, salt, and potato) along with vegetables, fruit, milk, tea, etc., that people consume daily in 3- or 4-course meals. Conventional food also includes such preserved foods as pickles and jams, bakery products, and yogurt. The term 'organic food' also comes under conventional food crops that are claimed to be produced by organic methods with no chemical fertilizers, pesticides, etc. applied at any stage. There are different variants of organic food available in the market but all are more expensive than the conventional foods, which are more widely available. Many brands have expanded their customer base by promoting their products as 100% organic, cruelty-free etc.; however, these claims are a matter of discussion.

Nutraceuticals are not conventional foods, but can be any of the five categories shown in Figure 4.

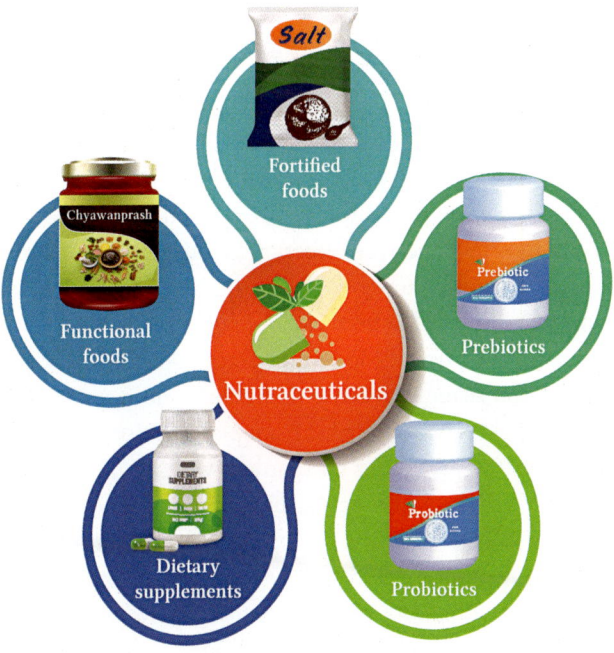

Figure 4 Types and examples of nutraceuticals in Indian market

Fortified foods are staple or conventional foods, the nutritional value of which has been increased by adding one or more nutrients, especially such key nutrients as minerals (iron and iodine, for example) and vitamins (A and D, for example). Such additions complement the original nutritional value of food and any loss that may have occurred in processing. The fortification is carried out in a way that maintains the original aroma and taste. Because these are staple foods, they are consumed by the majority and thus offer an easy way to overcome malnutrition. It has also been shown by the Copenhagen Consensus that fortified foods have a high benefit-to-cost ratio. Fortified foods commonly available in India are wheat flour and rice (fortified with iron, folic acid and vitamin B_{12}), salt (with iron and iodine), edible oils and milk (with vitamins A and D). Vita milk, Tata salt plus, Aashirvad aata, Fortune edible oil, and Daawat Sehat mogra are some commonly used fortified food brands in India.

Functional foods overlap with the conventional and fortified foods in many aspects and, in a nutshell, comprise food and food ingredients that provide additional health benefits along with the nutrients supplied by conventional food. Functional food is also defined as 'whole food with fortified, enriched, or enhanced foods that have potential beneficial effect on health when consumed as a part of a varied diet on a regular basis' (Crowe and Francis 2013). Chyavanprash is an old-school example of a functional food. The constituents of functional food range from macronutrients and essential micronutrients to those that are not nutrients at all, such as 'bioactive's, which are derived from plants, microorganisms, marine organisms, and other inorganic raw materials (Hasler and Brown 2009; Crowe and Francis 2013). *Ashwagandha (Withania somnifera,* an evergreen shrub), *giloy (Tinospora cordifolia,* a woody climber), *brahmi (Bacopa monnieri,* a perennial creeper), *and other medicinal plants also come under functional foods.*

Fortified and functional foods are broadly similar, as are the laws and regulations that apply to them.

Dietary supplements are supplements in the form of tablets, syrups, capsules, etc., that complement regular foods and typically include one or more minerals, vitamins, amino acids, extract of a herb or other botanical constituent, a bioactive metabolite, or any other dietary substance. These constituents can be in the form of a concentrate, an extract, or combinations of these ingredients. Dietary supplements are merely add-ons to ensure a balanced diet. The most commonly used supplements are multivitamins, calcium, protein powder, omega-3 capsules, and fish oil capsules. Omega-3 fatty acids are essential fatty acids that our bodies cannot synthesize and therefore must be provided through the diet (Spector and Kim 2015). Herbal dietary supplements are mixtures of various herbs converted into tonics or capsules taking into consideration the RDA (recommended dietary allowances). Spirulina powder or triphala powder come under this category.

Probiotics are nutraceuticals specifically aimed at ensuring that our gut harbours beneficial microorganisms that improve gut health. Prebiotics are non-digestible food ingredients that selectively stimulate the growth and activities of probiotic life forms, namely the beneficial bacteria that live in the colon. The Food Safety and Standards regulations, which are part of the act referred to earlier, put into effect some provisions from 1 April 2022. According to these provisions, "Prebiotic food means food that contains added ingredients which are non-viable food components that confer health benefits to the consumer by modulation of gut microbiota" and "Probiotic food means food with live micro-organisms beneficial to human health, which when ingested in adequate numbers as a single strain or as a combination of cultures, confer one or more specified or demonstrated health benefits in human beings."

The gut bacteria help in breaking down and digesting food, communicating with the immune system, keeping inflammation at bay, and in many more ways.

Given their essential role in maintaining stomach health, prebiotics and probiotics are widely used along with the prescribed medicines such as antibiotics. Probiotics are made specifically for the human gut so that they survive in the stomach and play roles similar to those of the gut bacteria. Prebiotics are a food source for the bacteria in intestinal tracts. As our digestive system cannot break them down, prebiotics pass through the tract and reach the colon, where they are consumed by bacteria for their nutrition and multiplication.

Instant nutrition products, or replacement meals, are designed for weight loss and hunger control or to deliver comprehensive nourishment to the time-starved generation with hectic schedules. Such products consist of powder mixes to be consumed after mixing with liquids such as water, milk, or juices; bars such as breakfast, protein, or energy bars; and other drinks.

Super foods are foods that are high in vitamins, minerals, antioxidants, and phytonutrients. Popular super foods include antioxidant-rich green vegetables such as spinach and broccoli, nuts high in phytosterols such as walnuts and almonds; fruit and vegetables with carotenoids such as carrots; and berries rich in polyphenols such as blueberries.

Some terms under the Food Safety and Standards Act

The Food Safety and Standards Act defines some terms under 'Health Supplements, Nutraceuticals, Foods for Special Dietary Uses, Foods for Special Medical Purposes and Prebiotic and Probiotic Foods Regulations, 2022', which are explained below.

Food for special medical needs is made especially to meet the nutritional requirements that are part of the treatment for a particular disease or condition or to mitigate its effects. Foods for special medical uses are specially processed or formulated for managing the diets of patients and may be used only under medical supervision. These foods are intended for the exclusive or partial feeding of patients with limited or impaired capacity to take, digest, absorb, or metabolize ordinary foodstuffs or some nutrients contained in such foodstuff or for those who have other special medically-determined nutritional requirements that cannot be met merely by modifying a normal diet. Such foods are to be sold only when prescribed and consumed only as advised by a physician following medical evaluation to establish the special nutritional requirements. Infant formulas and some ready-to-use foods are the most common examples of medical foods. These foods are intended to affect the structure or function of the body and initially classified as drugs. Before commercial release as a pharmaceutical drug, such foods have to undergo proper preclinical and clinical trials. We commonly encounter such foods in hospitals and are administered through a nasogastric tube to those who are unable to eat the normal diet (patients recovering from a surgery, for example). Ready-to-use therapeutic foods are used because they can be consumed directly without any cooking or preparation and provide a set quantity of every required nutrient as part of the recommended dietary allowance. Special medical foods do not make any particular claims but are merely formulas to meet nutritional requirements and are made from fruits, vegetables, meat, dairy, cereals, etc.

Bioactives are chemical compounds that are not directly involved in growth but are responsible for effects, responses, or reactions in living beings. Carbohydrates, fatty acids, peptides, etc., in concentrated forms come under bioactives and are obtained from various sources including plants, mushrooms, animals, and microorganisms and help in normal regulation of bodily functions. Antioxidative, anti-inflammatory, and antimicrobial activities of curcumin present in turmeric or carotenoids present in fruit are among the important applications of bioactives.

Foods for special dietary use are specially processed or formulated foods that are designed to satisfy specific dietary requirements arising from a particular physical or physiological condition or specific diseases and disorders. The composition of these foodstuffs must differ significantly from the composition of ordinary foods, if any, of comparable nature. Foods for special dietary uses are intended to be used as adjuncts to the management of diseases or disorders and only under medical prescription and supervision.

Sources of nutraceuticals

The most common source of nutraceuticals is plants. Products obtained from plants make up a significant part of our daily meals. Food grains, vegetables, fruits, and spices are the primary constituents of conventional or functional food. These products are the treasure box of nutrition. Another important source is products of animal origin, which include milk and milk products, fish, and meat products. Table 2 lists some sources of nutraceuticals.

> **Box 4 Some key terms defined**
>
> Recommended dietary allowance is the average daily intake of food sufficient to meet the nutritional requirements of nearly all (97%–98%) healthy people.
>
> Organic food is food grown or raised without the use of additives, colouring, synthetic chemicals (such as fertilizers, pesticides, and hormones), radiation, or genetic manipulation and meeting the criteria stipulated by the US Department of Agriculture's Standard National Organic Program.
>
> Bioactives are compounds responsible for biological properties other than normal physiological actions.
>
> Omega 3-fatty acids are a group of polyunsaturated fatty acids that are important for a number of functions in the body.
>
> Pharmaceutical drugs, also called medication or medicines, are chemical substances used for the treatment, cure, prevention, or diagnosis of a disease or to promote well-being.

Table 2 Sources of different types of nutraceuticals

Source	Product	Type of nutraceutical
Plants		
Bioactives	Phytochemicals	Bioactives
Cereals	Rice fortified with iron and vitamin B_{12}	Fortified foods
Fruits and nuts	Vitamins, minerals, antioxidants	Dietary supplements
Medicinal herbs	Antioxidants, immuno-boosters, macronutrients	Functional foods, bioactives
Spices	Anti-diabetic, anti-inflammatory products	Bioactives, functional foods, dietary supplements
Vegetables	All nutrients	Bioactives, dietary supplement, fortified food, functional foods
Animals		
Dairy products	Protein, lactose derivatives, vitamins, minerals, probiotics, prebiotics	Fortified food, dietary supplement, bioactives
Meat	Proteins, fatty acids, minerals, vitamins	Dietary supplements, functional foods, fortified foods
Sea food	Fatty acids, minerals, carbohydrates	Bioactives, dietary supplements
Microorganisms		
Bacteria	Lactobacillus, gut bacteria	Probiotics, bioactives
Micro algae	Spirulina, Chlorella	Probiotics, dietary supplements

What is in our food supplements
Consumer awareness and regulations
The global use of nutraceuticals has increased immensely in the last decade and especially during the COVID-19 pandemic when vitamins and minerals supplements were being prescribed routinely by doctors. As consumption of nutraceuticals is considered a preventive measure with less to no side effects if taken correctly, the nutraceuticals market has seen good growth. With a number of brands and different types of products in the market, consumers find it difficult to decide what are the right nutraceuticals for them.

Now that we have a broad idea of what nutraceuticals are and why we use them, the next important aspect to consider is how to use them effectively to get the most out of them. Smart phones offer a perfect analogy: one can use them far more effectively if one knows all their functions fully.

Labelling categories and claims
Labels for food supplements, as those for foods, must list all the constituents. The label for vitamins and minerals must specify the amount of each nutrient per serving as well as the per cent DV (percentage daily value) of the serving as a proportion of the recommended dietary allowance. Other dietary supplements such as botanicals (herbs) must include the amount per serving as well as the plant organ (root, leaves, and so on) from which the component is derived. The weights of each component that makes up a manufacturer's unique blend of two or more components (e.g., botanicals) must be listed (Figure 5).

Regulations laid down by the FSSAI (https://fssai.gov.in/upload/uploadfiles/files/FOOD-ACT.pdf) stipulate the following labelling requirements for nutraceuticals.
- The labelling or presentation must not claim that the nutraceutical product has the property of preventing, curing or treating human disease. It must not even make reference to any such properties.

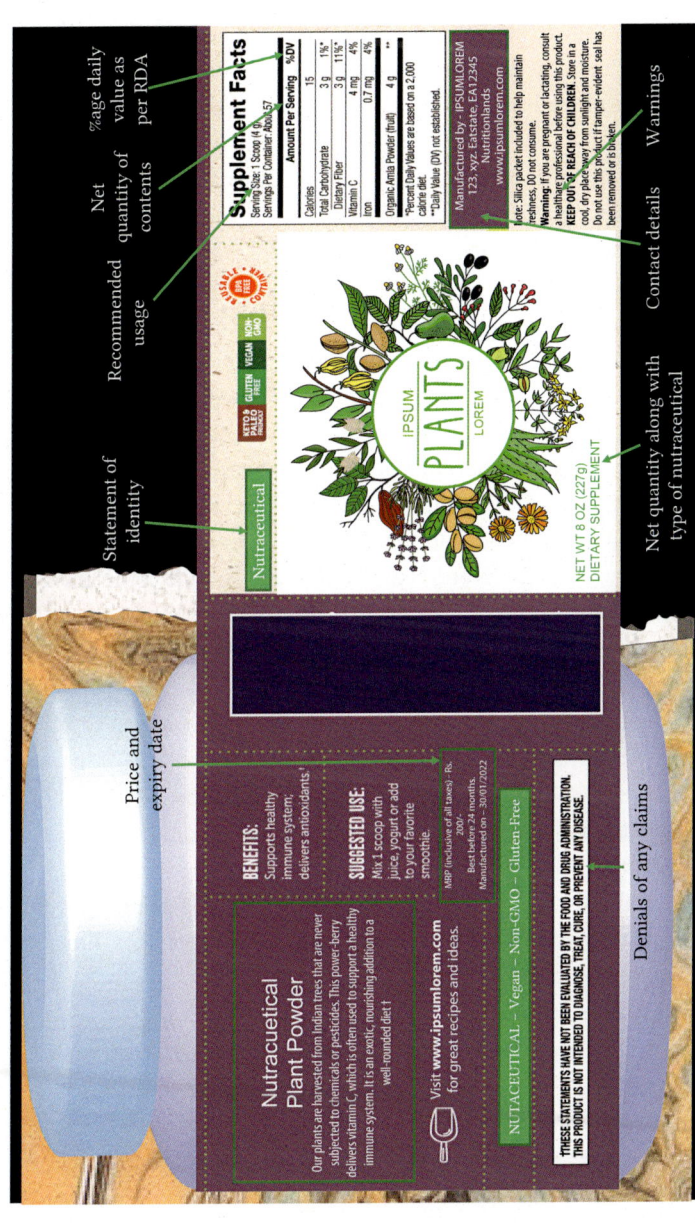

Figure 5 A consumer-friendly supplement label

- The food authority will allow such statements only if the statement made by the brand regarding the structure or function or the general well-being of the body is supported by scientific evidence.
- Every package of food containing nutraceuticals shall carry the following information on the label.
  — The word 'nutraceutical'
  — The common name of the nutraceutical
  — A declaration about the amount of each nutraceutical ingredient in the product that has either a nutritional or physiological value.
  — When nutrients are added, it must be mentioned along with its quantity expressed in terms of percentage of the RDA as specified by the Indian Council of Medical Research even if the nutrients are in addition to a nutraceutical, and the label shall bear an advisory warning 'Not to exceed the stated recommended daily usage'.
  — An advisory warning 'Not for medicinal use' should be prominently written
  — An advisory warning in case of possible danger from excessive consumption
  — An advisory warning or any other warning or precaution to be taken while consuming, known side effects, contraindications, and product–drug interactions, as applicable
  — A statement that the product is required to be stored out of reach of children
  — Nutritional information or nutritional facts per 100 grams or 100 millilitres or per serving of the product shall be given on the label containing the following details.
    - Energy value, in kcal
    - The amounts of protein, carbohydrate (specify quantity of sugar) and fat, in grams (g)
    - The amount of any other nutrient for which a nutrition- or health-related claim is made provided that if a claim is made regarding the amount or type of fatty acids or the amount of cholesterol, the amount of saturated fatty acids, mono-unsaturated fatty acids, and polyunsaturated fatty acids

in grams (g) and cholesterol in milligrams (mg) shall be declared, and the amount of trans fatty acid in grams (g) shall be declared in addition to the other requirement stipulated above.
- Wherever numerical information on vitamins and minerals is declared, it shall be expressed in metric units.
- Where the nutrition declaration is made per serving, the amount in grams (g) or millilitres (mL) shall be included for reference beside the serving measure.

In addition, nutraceuticals must have the following information too on the label as prescribed by the Legal Metrology Packaged Commodities Rules, 2011, as they are a packaged commodity.

- The common or generic names of the commodity must be mentioned on the label and if the commodity has more than one product, the name and the quantity of each product must be mentioned.
- The net quantity or the number of the commodity must be mentioned.
- Information on 'best before' or 'use by', that is the expiry date, must be mentioned on the label lest the product should become unfit for human consumption.
- The retail sale price of the package.
- Where the size of the packages is an important feature, the dimensions of the commodity must be mentioned.
- It must be ensured that each package bears the name, address, telephone number, and e-mail address of the person or office to be contacted in case of consumer complaints.
- It is not permissible to affix individual stickers on the package for making any declaration or altering it under these rules.
- Where the commodity consists of a number of components packed in units to be sold as a single commodity, the declarations must be made on the main package or such declaration must be given on individual packages and intimation of the same shall be given on the main package.

How to read a label

We are all familiar with the ingredients section in the labels of packaged foods although the terms are usually difficult to interpret. Dividing these terms into different categories gives us some idea of what we would be consuming and how we should consume it. The supplementary facts in Figure 5 can be taken as an example.

First, the serving size is mentioned, given in terms of, for example, a scoop (supplied with the food) or a teaspoon, etc., for powders or liquids or the number of tablets, along with the total number of servings that can be obtained from the quantity supplied.

Next is a list of ingredients, typically divided into three columns, namely the ingredient, amount per serving, and the percentage of dietary value. The ingredients are nutrients (carbohydrates, fats, etc., the number of calories, and any chemical or any plant extract added to the formulation); the amount per serving is the amount of each ingredient present in one serving (one scoop, one tablet, one teaspoon, or whatever); and the percentage of dietary value, or % DV, is the proportion of the RDA present in one serving taking into consideration the average calorie intake. For example, if the recommended dietary value of carbohydrates is 300 g a day for an individual taking a 2000-calorie diet and the %DV is 1%, it means that one serving contains 3 grams of carbohydrates.

When we take any nutraceutical that claims to be a nutritional supplement, we should make sure that the %DV is not too high when taken in addition to our normal diet because excess may prove toxic. At the same time, the percentage should not be so low that the purpose of taking a supplement is not served. Therefore, it is important to take into account the supplements and the diet prescribed by a physician or a health expert before adding, discontinuing, or changing the supplement.

Lastly, the label also tells us how many servings must be taken in a day. If more than the prescribed amount is taken, it can create imbalance in the daily nutrient intake and, in severe cases, can lead to nutrient toxicity. And if we take less than the prescribed amount, the supplement may not give the desired results.

Regulations and false claims

Section 23 (Packaging and Labelling Foods) of the FSSAI regulations offers the following guidelines related to the claims made by any nutraceutical.

(1) No person shall manufacture, distribute, sell or expose for sale or dispatch or deliver to any agent or broker for the purpose of sale, any packaged food products which are not marked and labelled in the manner as may be specified by regulations.

The labels shall not contain any statement, claim, design or device which is false or misleading in any particular concerning the food products contained in the package or concerning the quantity or the nutritive value implying medicinal or therapeutic claims or in relation to the place of origin of the said food products.

(2) Every food business operator shall ensure that the labelling and presentation of food, including their shape, appearance or packaging, the packaging materials used, the manner in which they are arranged and the setting in which they are displayed, and the information which is made available about them through whatever medium, does not mislead consumers.

Other provisions in the regulations allow products to be analysed and inspected; those that found unsafe or about which false claims are made in advertisements can be cancelled and their manufacturers can be punished. Section 24 ('Restrictions of advertisement and prohibition as to unfair trade practices') of the regulations includes the following provisions.

- No advertisement shall be made of any food that is misleading or deceiving or contravenes the provisions of this act, and the rules and regulations included in it.
- No person shall engage in any unfair trade practice for the purpose of promoting the sale, supply, use, or consumption of articles

of food or adopt any unfair or deceptive practice including the practice of making any statement, whether orally or in writing or by visible representation that

— (a) falsely represents that the foods are of a particular standard, quality, quantity or grade-composition;

— (b) makes a false or misleading representation concerning the need for, or the usefulness of; or

— (c) gives to the public any guarantee of the efficacy that is not based on adequate or scientific justification thereof,

provided that where a defence is raised to the effect that such guarantee is based on adequate or scientific justification, the burden of proof of such defence shall lie on the person raising such defence.

Section 2 (1) (r) of the existing Consumer Protection Act, 1986, states that the practice of making any statement, whether orally or in writing or by visible representation that falsely represents that the goods are of a particular standard, quality, quantity, grade, composition style or model or falsely represents that the services are of a particular standard, quality or grade, falls under unfair trade practices.

Marketing gimmicks versus realities

A study conducted by the Associated Chambers of Commerce and Industry of India in 2015 found 60%–70% of food supplements sold in India, a two-billion-dollar industry, to be counterfeit, unregistered, and unapproved (https://medium.com/sparxchain/fake-nutraceuticals-a-global-health-and-economic-concern-52327ba04907). In a few cases, the regulations were not properly followed. Many nutraceutical formulations are marketed as over-the-counter drugs in local pharmacies. These formulations might be beneficial and can be used without a medical prescription. For example, the extract of grape seeds is claimed to have anti-inflammatory properties: although the claim is backed by no valid data, the extract it can be given as an over-the-counter drug by a chemist if a customer wishes to buy it. However, some formulations, if given without proper examination or consultation can be toxic or cause an otherwise adverse reaction. Also, without a diagnosis, any drug or supplement can be a potential poison in a matter of minutes although the lay public is misled into thinking that it can cure a particular malady.

Pharmaceuticals versus nutraceuticals

Pharmaceuticals are drugs that are used only after they are prescribed by a medical practitioner for the treatment, control, or detection of a disease or disorder. Such drugs generally go through rigorous tests and strict trials as governed by the regulatory framework of the Drugs and Cosmetics Act, 1945. Pharmaceuticals are derived mainly from chemicals including minerals and electrolytes and developed following a thorough literature search, hundreds of bioinformatical and laboratory analyses; undergo various tests to identify their efficacy, non-lethal dosage, and reactions with other drugs or chemicals and then undergo trials on various living systems and are accepted only if they give consistently reproducible and stable results. The drugs then reach human trials with a good amount of data proving their safety after years of research. Drugs also generally target a particular disease or condition and therefore not available immediately to treat a previously unknown disease (for example plague, as virus like Ebola, Spanish Flu, or COVID-19) and cannot be used for treating such diseases until a drug is proven safe, effective, and non-toxic. The discovery of penicillin as an antibacterial drug or of insulin to treat diabetes made a history and now forms part of the school curriculum. Banning of thalidomide because it led to defects in the newborn and of methamphetamine because it was abused as a narcotic also revolutionized every country's regulations governing the development and testing of drugs. Another angle is that drugs mostly consist of only one active ingredient or a combination of more than one in fixed proportions and in adequate amounts and a few other common ingredients to make drugs more acceptable to patients. Drug labels always give information about any interactions a drug might have with other drugs or food ingredients, how the drug works, and what one should take or do – or avoid taking or doing – to make the drug more effective.

Nutraceuticals, on the other hand, are not that difficult to introduce in the market once a certain property in an extract or component is identified. Data are collected based on the solubility, toxicity levels, formulations, and stability in the selected form. The nutraceutical can be in the form of a tablet, syrup, or powder and tested on far fewer individuals than those involved in testing pharmaceuticals. The general procedure for getting a license for releasing a nutraceutical in the market includes adding details of the product in the Food Product Identity Verification System (Figure 6): it is checked if the product falls in any of the standard product categories and if it does, the product is given a product identifier, generated automatically, which helps in obtaining a license from the appropriate licensing authority. The Food Safety and Standards Authority of India checks whether the information on the label meets the Food Safety & Standards (Packaging & Labelling) Regulations, 2011. The chemical, physical, and biological properties of the product are then analysed following appropriate guidelines and, if the results of the analysis are acceptable, a license is issued (https://foodsafetyhelpline.com/fssai-registration-licensing-and-compliance-for-nutraceuticalshealth-suppliments/). The process generally takes roughly 2–3 years and is therefore far quicker than that in the case of pharmaceuticals. This major difference between pharmaceuticals and nutraceuticals is the main reason nutraceuticals are not considered drugs or medicines and can replace neither medicines nor food.

Current market space for nutraceuticals

Nutraceuticals are produced mainly by pharmaceuticals, FMCG (fast moving consumer goods) companies worldwide, and a few pure-play nutraceutical companies. These research-backed innovative companies introduce products in the market quite frequently because they have designated R&D departments that work on the formulations for new products. These companies have managed to place such nutraceuticals as fortified foods, dietary supplements, and functional foods and beverages on shop shelves and home cabinets. Functional beverages, similar to functional foods, are beverages that provide additional health benefits along with their normal nutritional value and include functional juices, malt-based drinks, energy beverages, prebiotic and probiotic drinks, functional ready-to-drink teas, alternative to dairy beverages, and water (water with vitamins, minerals, acids, herbs, raw fruits or vegetables, etc.).

Global trends in a nutshell

It is not surprising that nutraceutical industries contribute to the global economy. The global nutraceuticals market was valued at about $455 billion in 2021 and is expected to grow at a CAGR (compound annual growth rate, or mean annual growth rate of an investment for a period longer than a year) of 9% from 2021 to 2030 (https://www.grandviewresearch.com/industry-analysis/nutraceuticals-market). The phenomenal growth can be attributed to the pandemic, as people began focusing on prevention and realized the importance of health. The United States, many European countries, and Japan account for 90% of the supplements market because of the increase in lifestyle-related diseases and sedentary living, as multivitamins and health supplements have become an integral part of the daily routine in those countries—which were also the first to regulate all types of nutraceuticals.

The Asia Pacific market – particularly China, India, Indonesia, and Malaysia – is also looking up, and the region is expected to witness significant growth from 2021 to 2030. India accounted for 2% of the global nutraceuticals market (valued at 4 billion dollars) by 2020, and Indian market is expected to grow at a CAGR of

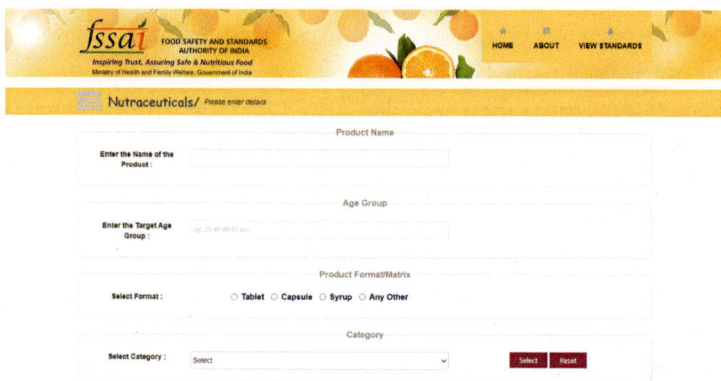

Figure 6 A screenshot of the food product identity verification system of the Food Safety and Standards Authority of India (https://fpas.fssai.gov.in/nutraceuticals)

21%, reaching 18 billion dollars by 2025 (Investor Portal, Ministry of Food Processing Industries). Many old FMCG companies have started to launch nutraceuticals and many new ones focusing exclusively on nutraceuticals have established a base in Indian market. With increasing acceptance of nutraceuticals by consumers, these new companies and products have been able to command attention and to build a good consumer base.

Indian scenario
Nutraceuticals based on herbal extracts including those of medicinal plants and spices have been used in India, China, and other Asian countries since ancient times, and the knowledge of their benefits has been passed down from generation to generation. India has been using commercialized nutraceuticals for some decades now. Baby foods, flavoured milk powders rich in vitamins and minerals, and iodized salt are among the most widely known fortified and functional foods in India. The major target of the nutraceuticals market in India are children, pregnant women, and the elderly. Malnutrition among children is rampant in India,

exacerbated by poverty and lack of clean food and water. The state has been active in alleviating malnutrition and has launched several schemes for the purpose, including Integrated Child Development Services, the National Health Mission, the mid-day meal scheme, and the *Poshan Abhiyan* (nutrition movement) of the central Ministry of Women and Child Development.

Problems due to an unhealthy lifestyle – obesity, for example – have become an everyday concern. Diet plans by physicians and fitness trainers mostly include nutraceuticals in the form of protein powders, energy drinks, etc. Calorie regulation is another aspect of diet that prompts people to use fortified and functional foods together with dietary supplements to ensure adequate nutrition but with fewer calories.

A report by the World Bank, titled *Nutrition in India*, estimates that India loses nearly 12 billion dollars of its GDP (gross domestic product) to malnourishment. However, interventions to alleviate the loss would cost merely about 524 million dollars annually—a benefit-to-cost ratio of almost 23. This focus on preventive care has also been strengthened by concerns over the increasing costs of health care: out-of-pocket expenses account for 62% of health care costs in India, and 60% of prescriptions in India include health and dietary supplements (https://www.investindia.gov.in/team-india-blogs/growing-nutraceuticals-market-india).

Nutraceuticals market and trade in India
India has the largest number of US FDA (Food Development Authority) approved plants located outside USA. India's infrastructure base and the 'make in India' policy of the Government of India has been attracting foreign investments in the sector. One hundred per cent FDI (foreign direct investment) is permitted in manufacturing of nutraceuticals. The investment helps in creating jobs with higher skills and superior technologies and also helps the stakeholders including farmers, traders, and retailers.

Several multinational and Indian companies have been promoting and selling nutraceuticals in India on a large scale and are trusted greatly by consumers. Exclusive outlets and brand endorsements by celebrities make the products more credible in consumers' eyes, and this has helped companies that manufacture fitness products to enter the market. Online health-supplement stores, pharmacies, and medical stores have made nutraceuticals easily available to consumers, and this easy availability has helped to create more opportunities for investment in e-commerce related aspects of the nutraceuticals market. Dietary supplements and functional food and beverages contribute a significant amount to Indian economy (Figure 7).

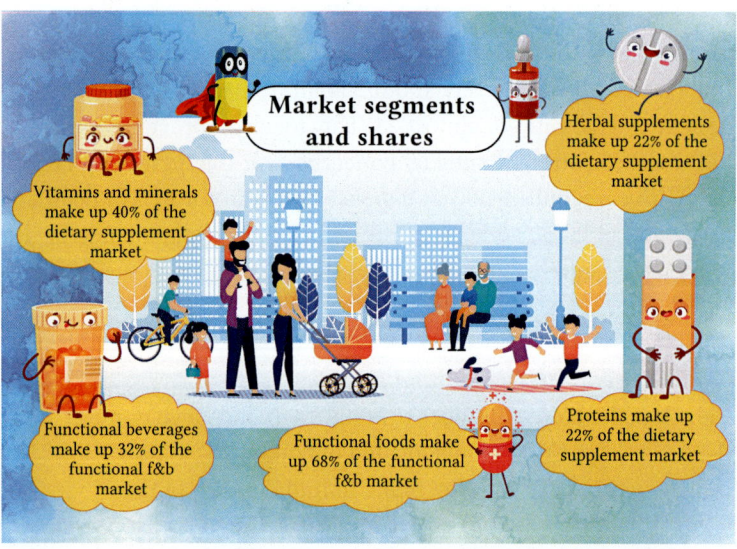

Figure 7 Shares of different dietary supplements, functional foods and beverages in Indian nutraceuticals market (**source** ASSOCHAM, Ministry of Food Processing Industries)

India is still in the developing phase in the nutraceuticals market and production, well behind such market leaders as the United States, Japan, and many European countries. However, attractive incentives and support from the Government of India and innovations from the R&D departments of Indian companies would soon create a powerful impact on the global market.

Major growth drivers of nutraceuticals market
Many factors contribute to the increased use of nutraceuticals, and some major ones are described below (Figure 8).

Communicable diseases are such infectious diseases as viral infections (COVID-19), plague, malaria, and hepatitis that can be transmitted from one person to another through body fluids, aerosols, contaminated surfaces, food, water, etc. The most recent pandemic is one such disease. Although such diseases can be prevented only by avoiding any contact with infected people, the immune response and the severity of the disease can vary depending on the individual. Those with a strong immune system and a healthy body will be less harmed by the infection than those who are poorly nourished and lack the nutrients even for the normal functions of the body. To use an analogy, a laptop equipped with proper anti-virus software and processor is more likely to combat a virus attack successfully than a laptop that can barely manage to keep five tables or windows open without hanging. The difference became increasingly obvious during the COVID-19 pandemic, encouraging many to shift to more nutritious and home-cooked food from fast food.

Non-communicable diseases (lifestyle and chronic) diseases are the ones which can be transferred from one person to other but appear due to genetic conditions, hereditary reasons or effects of lifestyle. Cardio-vascular diseases constitute the major part of deaths caused by non-communicable diseases followed by chronic respiratory disorders, cancers, diabetes and others. Eating fat-rich and high-cholesterol oily foods, not having enough food, obesity,

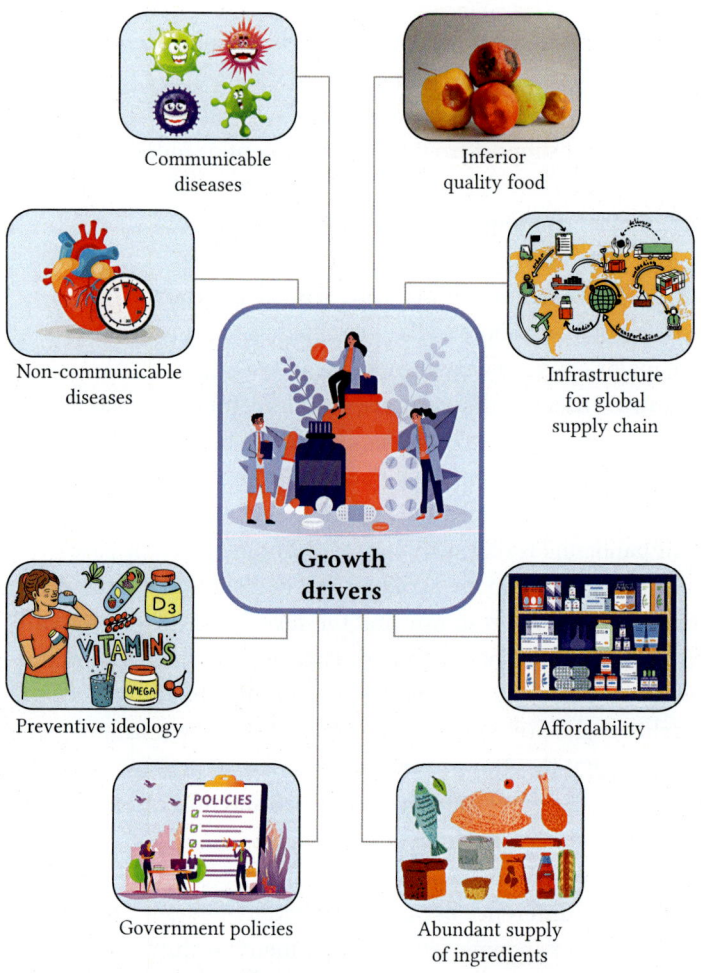

Figure **8** Some key growth drivers leading the booming nutraceuticals market in India

sedentary living, and many more are the major reasons why these diseases cause more deaths than any other factor. Even if the disease is run in family, getting a proper nutritious food with some physical activity can help the individual to supress it to some extent. Not having a complete nutrition can lead to resurfacing of the disease even after treatments.

Inferior quality of food produced by modern industrial-scale farming may require nutraceuticals to compensate for the low quality. Extensive use of chemical pesticides and fertilizers, cultivating the same crop year after year on the same plot of land, and preservative coating to prolong the shelf life of produce and to make it glossy and more appealing are among the practices that make such food not only somewhat unsafe but also less nutritious. Organic food, which is claimed to be chemical free, is expensive and not easily available. Therefore, even a seemingly balanced diet may not provide adequate nutrition—and nutraceuticals step in to make up the loss.

Increased emphasis on disease prevention has made nutraceuticals particularly popular. The realization that viral infections can prove less severe to those with healthy diets or with stronger immunity – claimed to be conferred by some nutraceuticals – has widened the market for them.

Greater affordability of nutraceuticals, especially when they are available in small sachets, makes them particularly appealing, readily available and easy to buy, herbal teas being a good example. Greater demand, economies of scale, and cheaper raw materials have made it possible for major FMCG companies to sell such nutraceuticals as fortified foods and functional foods at affordable prices and yet make a profit. Such fortified foods mean that more and more consumers now incorporate calcium or iron in the diet of their children.

Extensive trade infrastructure to meet the demands of global supply chains have facilitated both imports and exports. With 7500 kilometres of coastline, 12 major ports, 200 minor ports, and 100 operational airports, India is well connected not only to almost all its neighbours but to the whole world. Nearly half of India's herbal products and approximately 13% of dietary supplements are exported.

Abundant supply of raw materials, namely fruit, vegetables, milk, food grains – India is a major producer of all of them – makes it easy to isolate nutrients from them, process the extracted nutrients, and convert them into concentrated forms.

Encouragement from the state has also boosted the nutraceuticals sector. As part of its 'make in India' policy, the Indian government wants to leverage India's position as the rising player in the global supply chain, reduce its imports of pharmaceuticals and encourage their manufacture in the country. The central Ministry of Food Processing Industries has set up a web portal (Figure 9) to attract investments in India's nutraceuticals market. This portal supplies details of the incentives offered by the state and of policies to support investments in the food processing industry.

Restorative concluding remarks

Nutraceuticals are consumed as a preventive measure and to improve health and can help people if taken at the right time and in the right amounts. They contribute to better health and can even delay the onset of adverse genetic conditions by maintaining the body's internal systems in good condition (Figure 10). Nutraceuticals are usually offered as concentrated nutrients

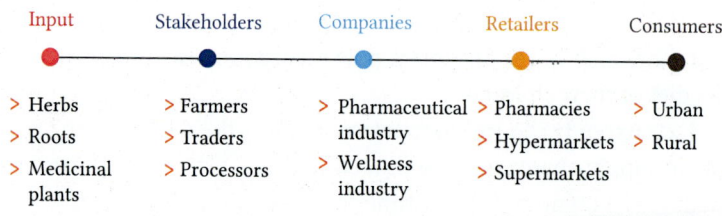

Figure **9** Value chain of nutraceuticals on the investor portal set up by the Ministry of Food Processing Industries (https://foodprocessingindia.gov.in/sectors/Nutraceuticals)

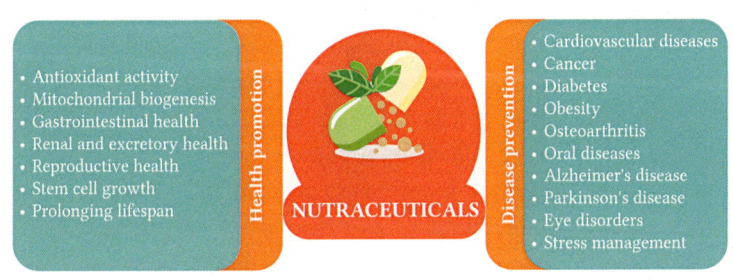

Figure **10** Role of nutraceuticals in maintaining well-being

in the form of small tablets that add no fat, sodium, or calories. However, nutraceuticals should not be taken as a 'replacement' for a normal diet. It is important to note that nutraceuticals work best when they complement the normal diet and pharmaceuticals. Sometimes people begin to consume more of nutraceuticals or start taking them more frequently because they feel energized after taking them—which then lose their efficacy. However, the effects vary depending on a person's state of health and heredity and physiological make-up. For example, products based on glucosamine-chondroitin are popular among those who suffer from arthritis, and many herbal teas and functional foods are useful to those with diabetes; these products have built a customer base over the past two decades. A significant market exists for products that can build immunity in children and in those who might be susceptible to infections or suffering from other effects of infective diseases.

Consuming nutraceuticals: frequently asked questions
Will conventional foods and a balanced diet without supplements or nutraceuticals meet all the nutritional needs for a long and healthy life?

A balanced diet contains all the nutrients that a human body needs for its normal functioning and for leading an emotionally and physically healthy life. Individuals differ in their body composition, age, gender, hereditary attributes, and medical history. Moreover, the environment, physical activity, and eating habits may also vary from person to person. For example, the dietary requirement of an athlete will differ from those of a person doing a 9-to-5 desk job. Meals should also vary with the season, lifestyle, medical advice (when required), and the psychological environment (stress inducing, neutral, or relaxing). All these factors play a role in controlling our cravings, meal schedules, and appetites and, in turn, the intake and absorption of nutrients.

If you can maintain proper levels of nutrients taking into consideration all the above and other relevant factors, you will be able to sustain a healthy life without taking supplements—nutraceuticals are for those who are unable to balance these factors.

I feel tired all the time and cannot perform even basic chores properly. I have checked these symptoms on the internet, and I think I suffer from iron or vitamin deficiency. Should I take multivitamins or iron tablets?

Self-diagnoses are common nowadays, especially with the resources available on internet in public domain. Chronic fatigue may have various underlying reasons including burnout from overwork, any mental health condition or recurring physical health condition or deficiency. A medical check-up is therefore advisable before you start taking any supplements on your own. Such a check-up may seem unnecessarily expensive but early diagnosis can save a lot of expenditure later. A professional can answer all your queries about your physical or mental health and will prescribe the right supplements if required.

For the past two months, I have been taking a protein supplement before working out and I have obtained quicker results and have never felt this good. Can I take more of the supplement for even better results?

One should not increase or decrease the dose of any supplement until recommended by a professional following a full check-up. Tempting as it may be to see a better physical version of you, being patient and consistent is the key. Be more cautious of what goes inside your body and how much. More of anything can be dangerous.

If I can get all my nutrients from supplements and medical foods without any extra calories or fat, why should I bother eating normal food? I can live on the supplements alone.

Natural foods derived from plants and animals are always the best and should be the first option for obtaining all the nutrients and compounds. Plants contain phytochemicals and some other compounds that play a role in the well-being of an individual but are missing from any nutraceuticals so far. All meals cannot be 'replaced' with nutraceuticals. Natural foods are safe and has hardly any side effects unless the wrong types of foods are mixed or adulterated or spoiled foods are consumed.

There is so much information on every single type of nutraceuticals and so many brands to choose from. What should be the best option for me?

Here is a handy checklist to help in choosing the safest and most efficient supplements.

- A well-known and FDA- or FSSAI-approved brand that has earned good customer reviews and carries the FSSAI license number (typically fresh products because the product is in constant demand)

- Date of expiry at least 3 months later than the day of purchase and product with a long shelf life
- Absence of any unrealistic claims (for example, 'Building muscles within a week') or claims of being 'natural' or 'organic' and therefore expensive—all nutrients are chemicals and function the same way irrespective of source if taken properly
- Clearly laid out and informative label (for example, whether refrigerated storage is essential)

How do I know whether the claims made for a product are true?
If a product supplies more than 20% of the daily recommended dietary allowance (%DV) per dose, the product is rich in that compound; if the corresponding figure is 5% or less, the content is low. For example, if a product claims to be rich in vitamins, check if it supplies more than 20% of the daily recommended intake—if it does not, the claim is false.

How do I compare the labels on different products to find out which one is better?
Here is a checklist to help you choose the type of nutraceutical or food supplement brand.
- Look at the list of ingredients or the composition to see if it mentions vitamins, minerals, fibre, proteins, or other nutrients and also check if you are allergic to any of these.
- Look for the FSSAI license number.
- See whether, and to what extent, the %DV of all the components meet your requirements.
- Carefully read all the warnings and precautions on the label to ensure that no warning or precaution poses a threat to any relevant medical condition.

Honest Abe's valuable advice
The best way to capture the role of supplements in good nutrition may be to paraphrase Abraham Lincoln's famous remark about

politicians and voters: "You may fool all the people some of the time; you can even fool some of the people all the time; but you can't fool all the people all the time." If Honest Abe were with us now and were a sensible nutritionist rather than a president, he might have put it thus: "Best to get your nutrients from food. Supplements are valuable for all people some of the time and for some people all the time, but they're probably not necessary for all people all the time."

Challenges for nutraceuticals

Some supplements can lead to various side effects. For example, garlic can increase the risk of bleeding in people taking blood thinners, and concentrated caffeine can be fatal. Such information should be mentioned on the labels and taken into consideration every time one buys a supplement.

Some companies sell supplements without proper testing. These supplements can have serious side effects. For example, ephedra is a herb and a supplement based on its extract was used for losing weight faster and for enhancing sports performance and also in traditional medicine to treat a cold, fever, or headache. The supplement was tested on a few people and released for sale. Later, it was reported that taking ephedra may also cause anxiety, dizziness, dry mouth, headache, irritability, nausea, personality changes, insomnia, and other symptoms (https://www.nccih.nih.gov/health/ephedra). With a prior medical condition or with any other stimulant such as caffeine, ephedra can cause severe conditions. Even then, it took the FDA at least 3 years to ban ephedra, because the FDA cannot compel a drug to be withdrawn until enough evidence of its ill effects is available.

Counterfeit products are a major challenge facing the nutraceutical industry. The most common method of counterfeiting in the nutraceuticals industry is undercutting the ingredients mentioned on the label, partly or fully, and replacing them with cheaper and easier-to-obtain alternatives.

The substitute ingredient is often undeclared in the claims, which proves risky for those allergic to it. Another form of adulteration is to add an active chemical pharmaceutical ingredient to improve the efficacy of the nutraceutical without declaring the ingredient on the label. A few companies promote their products as being of natural origin, but add chemicals to achieve the therapeutic effect claimed. Because companies licensed to manufacture nutraceuticals do not need to get product approvals unless they are working with new ingredients that are not part of the approved list, it is hard to nip the problem of adulterated products in the bud before they reach the market. Thus, despite consistent efforts by government authorities and a fair number of companies that adhere to regulations, the few dishonest companies damage the reputation of the industry as a whole.

E-commerce in India is growing exponentially all consumer products, including pharmaceuticals and nutraceuticals. E-pharmacies as well as direct sale to consumers through company e-stores have become increasingly common, and many manufacturers with reputable and credible products use online distribution channels to deliver directly to the end user at competitive prices. However, regulatory supervision is far lower in e-retail, and ethical manufacturers are often overshadowed by fraudulent companies with spurious products. Whereas e-pharmacies are becoming increasingly stringent for pharma products and make it mandatory for consumers to upload the relevant prescription for prescription drugs, the same level of control is not feasible for nutraceuticals, because most of them are in the OTC (over the counter) category.

Final remarks: individual-centric approach to nutraceuticals

Individual-centred approach is the only way to consume nutraceuticals. This approach is based on an individual's personal choices, behaviours, health status, genetic make-up, and the surrounding environment and also followed by physicians in prescribing nutraceuticals after assessing a person's nutritional requirements. A nutraceutical formulation (a combination of the nutrients missing or in low quantities in that individual) is then prescribed and should be taken only in the recommended dose and only for the prescribed duration. Normally, for any prescription, the diet and other intakes are taken into consideration lest anything in the diet should have a harmful reaction with the prescribed drugs or nutraceuticals leading to life-threatening incidents. Even plant-based botanicals or health supplements can have such adverse reactions. In most cases, the effects – fatigue, nausea, or headache, for example – are not serious although adverse effects such as a damaged liver and oxidative stress have also been reported.

The nutraceuticals market in India continues to attract investments from multinational companies and researchers. Companies have begun to realize that unvalidated products that are ineffective could affect the overall brand value and the company's image in the long term. Consumer awareness is also fuelling the effort to introduce new products, and supplements have moved from the standard heart health or liver health supplements to more niche areas. With increasing access to and advances in technology and the growing scientific understanding of plants and their extracts, coupled with globally evolving regulations and labelling guidelines for natural and organic certifications for home care and personal care products, a budding export market is opening up for natural herbal extracts made in India.

Bibliography

Brower V. 1998. Nutraceuticals: poised for a healthy slice of the healthcare market? *Nature Biotechnology* **16**: 728–731

Crowe K M, Francis C, and Academy of Nutrition and Dietetics. 2013. Position of the academy of nutrition and dietetics: functional foods. *Journal of the Academy of Nutrition and Dietetics* **113**: 1096–1103

DeFelice S L. 1995. The nutraceutical revolution: its impact on food industry R&D. *Trends in Food Science and Technology* **6**: 59–61

Gaynes R. 2017. The discovery of penicillin: new insights after more than 75 years of clinical use. *Emerging Infectious Diseases* **23**: 849–853

Hasler C M and Brown A C. 2009. Position of the American Dietetic Association: functional foods. *Journal of the American Dietetic Association* **109**: 735–746

Kim J H and Scialli A R. 2011. Thalidomide: the tragedy of birth defects and the effective treatment of disease. *Toxicological Sciences* **122**: 1–6. [Erratum in *Toxicological Sciences* **125**: 613]

NIDA. 2019. Methamphetamine DrugFacts. National Institute on Drug Abuse

Spector A A and Kim H Y. 2015. Discovery of essential fatty acids. *Journal of Lipid Research* **56**: 11–21

Vecchio I, Tornali C, Bragazzi N L, Martini M. 2018. The discovery of insulin: an important milestone in the history of medicine. *Frontiers in Endocrinology* **9**: 613 [8 pp.]

Zeisel S H. 1999. Regulation of "Nutraceuticals". *Science* **285**: 1853–1855

Some useful websites

European Nutrition Association https://www.enaonline.eu/

Food Safety and Standards Authority of India https://fssai.gov.in

Indian Council of Medical Research, National Institute of Nutrition https://www.nin.res.in/

National Health Portal https://www.nhp.gov.in/

US Dietary Supplement Health and Education Act, 1994 https://www.fda.gov/food/dietary-supplements